Tears
in My
Pocket

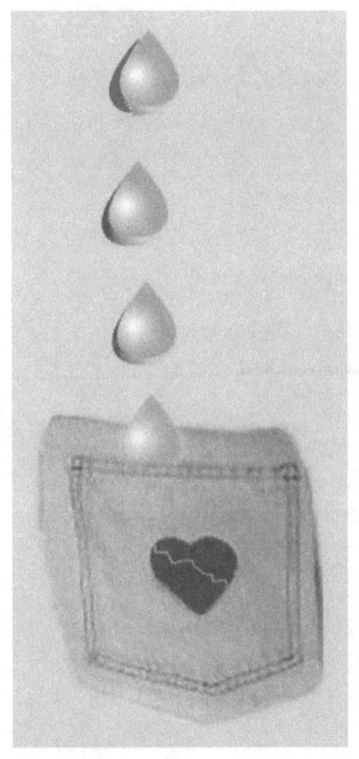

Sharon J. Hoffman

Order this book online at www.trafford.com
or email orders@trafford.com

Most Trafford titles are also available at major online book retailers.

Printed in the United States of America.

ISBN: 978-1-4269-6422-0 (sc)
ISBN: 978-1-4269-6423-7 (e)

Trafford rev. 04/13/2011

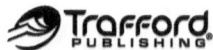

www.trafford.com

North America & international
toll-free: 1 888 232 4444 (USA & Canada)
phone: 250 383 6864 ♦ fax: 812 355 4082

Tears In My Pocket

Ten years ago, life changed drastically and forever. My husband and best friend of 36 years was diagnosed with lung cancer and five short months later, died.

With Larry's disease running rampant and all the while our options dwindled, until it finally came to a close on May 30, 2000.

I looked everywhere for answers.

First the library; then the computer; and even grief support.

For me, nothing I was searching for, was available.

Sure, I found statistics written by doctors or counselors, but I was searching for actual people who had experiences to share.

When the information I found, wasn't helpful or even sufficient, I knew I had to document my own experiences as I lived them day by day.

I was hoping to gather some insight along the way and maybe--just maybe help myself and possibly others who also were searching for answers to all the plaguing questions they had, and feelings they were experiencing.

I thought I was going crazy; that I was the only one thinking weird thoughts and behaving strangely. I found out that people who suffer losses of all kinds, sometimes do things that others may think bizarre.

I slept in Larry's pajamas; shared my bed with his box of ashes so 'he' would be close. I eventually put his pajamas on a body pillow so I could have something to snuggle up to.

Every night I'd kiss his 'box' and soon noticed that my tears had worn away some of the brass, that the box was made of.

Why does the word "Widow" bother me so much?

Maybe because it seems to label one.

Here is a person who no longer has a spouse. A person alone; a person grieving; a person to be pitied; a person no longer married but not single.

Whoa! That one really bothers me.

I'm still married. My partner died, I didn't.

I didn't chose to divorce nor choose to be single.

I wasn't given any choice at all!!!

I am still a married person whose spouse is no longer living with me, but not by choice.

Society labels people. "Golf widows" or "Football widows".

I never understood that. Just because a spouse is away from home, does not make their spouse a "widow".

Apparantly society has no idea what a "widow" is!

Is a person a "widow" if their spouse is away in the military?

How about if they're an Astronaut? Then, they aren't even on the planet.

I married till the end of my life and my life is not over.

If a person's spouse dies and they eventually remarry, then they are re-married.

If, like myself, I choose not to remarry; I am still married but alone, not single, which denotes available and unmarried.

I guess it is a personal definition, but to understand "my" premise to this book, you must understand it, from "my" definition.

Don't expect this to be an ordinary book.

I walk to a different beat and therefore this will probably be a book with a different slant on loss, grief and endurance.

It is however, reality; some may think I haven't moved forward.

Those will be the people who haven't experienced devastating loss to the degree I defined it.

Continuing---.

So, I eventually moved the box of cremains to the nightstand where it remains to this day.

Three and a half years after my husband died, my cat Missy also died.

She had been my only companion and now the sound of total silence was deafening. I never thought quiet could be so loud.

I had to have some noise, whether it be my radio or television.

Before, I was content with Missy's companionship and her gentle purring.

It was a nice, soothing sound and meant that I wasn't totally alone.

There was still life in the house and I could talk and interact with her.

When Missy died, I had her also cremated and now, her box sits atop Larrys box, on the nightstand.

It's comforting to know they're still close to me, and each other.

I talk to them and share my day with them.

When I leave the hosue, I say goodbye and upon my return, I yell out, "Hi honey, I'm home".

I don't kid myself. I know I'm alone. Just habit? Maybe.

Mental gymnastics? Whatever it is, it makes me feel connected somehow.

Chapter One — The Beginning

November 10, 1999

Larry and I set out on a trip back East and everything seemed fine.

He'd been a little tired. He developed what we thought was Laryngitis, so I had him gargle as I was a little concerned about it.

As we traveled and drove a long time, he would want to stop early each night. He wasn't hungry either. We just thought it was possible a cold was coming on with the Laryngitis. He kept asking me how long it was going to last. I told him, to my knowledge, Laryngitis could last about 7-10 days, but usually not as long as a cold.

But, being Larry, it would probably be a bit longer. He was stubborn and not liking to go to doctors or take medicine; letting things run their course could make it last long.

We continued to visit family and go to Antique Malls.

We really enjoyed each other and the time away.

It had been a long time since we had been able to get away by ourselves.

This Laryngitis thing went on all through the trip.

It began to get worse and eventually took a great toll on his voice.

It became very difficult for him to even talk above a whisper.
He seemed to have more residual problems; it just took his appetite completely away. Sometimes we'd start out at 7 AM and we wouldn't stop for anything to eat until about 5 or 6 PM, and then only because he thought I might be hungry.

We tried to stop at Cracker Barrel because it was one of his favorite places and I hoped it would stimulate his appetite.

We didn't know if anything was seriously going on, but it was perplexing that this 'laryngitis' thing was hanging on so long.

There were no special side effects. He didn't have a cough, fever or sore throat; it was just this laryngitis thing.

Trying to recap.

We took about a month for the trip and returned home about December 5th.

I was quite worried at that point, for this ailment had gone on too long, as far as I was concerned, and now I wanted him to see a doctor.

We were just in the middle of changing HMO doctors, as our current clinic was shutting down and transferring everything. They didn't have Larry's medical records at the new doctors office so I tried to fill them in as much as I could verbally, and say, "I want this checked out".

We went to our new Doctors office and the Primary physician was not available, so they gave us a P.A. (Physicians Assistant).

I don't hold her responsible in any way. The fact was; the P.A. didn't expect to find anything but routine conditions, unless he had a pre-existing condition that might have developed into something more serious. So, she wasn't looking for that to be the case.

She came into the examining room and I told her, we thought he had Laryngitis. I knew him well as we'd been married almost 36 years.

She kept saying that she thought he had a Sinus infection. I knew he did not. He had a Sinus infection about 20 years prior and the symptoms were totally different and unrelated to this. He wasn't having headaches, face pain, drainage and didn't react in the same way as a Sinus related condition.

But, not being a doctor myself; I couldn't reliably tell her she may be wrong, as she had to make a diagnosis herself, from her own observation.

[I might note: a bit of concern on my part as the P.A. never took Larry's blood pressure, temperature or even looked down his throat, which I thought was unusual].

She then proceeded to prescribe Sinus medication and an Antibiotic (only after looking in her *PDR for one)* Physicians Desk Reference.

I did go to the Pharmacy and had the prescriptions filled though knew in my heart it wouldn't do any good, and it didn't.

I finally decided enough was enough and it had gone 7 days, getting increasingly worse and Larry was getting much weaker. Now he was developing a soreness in his throat. I called back to the doctor's office and told them it wasn't working and that I didn't believe it was a Sinus infection. I asked to be referred to an ENT. (Ear, Nose & Throat)

I knew they would search more thoroughly and we definitely need something more conclusive.

I made an appointment and made it as urgent as possible.

We were taken in 2 days later and the doctor inserted a tube with a light connected, into Larry's throat and looked down into his Larynx.

He said he saw that there was something that needed more attention than he could give it.

He wrote a referral and sent us over to the hospital to have x-rays taken.

That was a bit worrisome for me but I really had no idea what could be going on.

I thought, "Let's not worry." "Let's wait and see; he's just covering all his bases."

The doctor's thoroughness somewhat reassured us at that point.

We arrived at the hospital and they took the x-rays. They told us to go home, which we did. The doctor would call for the results later on, and then inform us. We returned home which was about an hours drive and there was a message on the answering machine. The message was, "Please return to the Dr's office as he doesn't give this information over the phone."

At that point I started to get very concerned, so we immediately did return and the doctor said that Larry did NOT have Laryngitis but, instead, he had a Paralyzed vocal cord.

My first question was, "What caused the paralysis?"

The doctor said, "there is a tumor encroaching on his vocal cord and his voice will probably never come back."

There wasn't a whole lot he knew to do. You couldn't remove it without total damage and causing muteness. We then had several trips back and forth to the hospital; went through a battery of tests; went to see a Thorasic Surgeon. They did more extensive testing.

X-rays, MRI's, CAT scans and blood work, as well as Pulmonary Function tests. They then ordered a Thorosentisis.

At that point I opted to leave the room. I couldn't bear to see Larry endure that with me in the room. They were to insert a needle into his back; into his lung and extract fluid.

After the test I went back into the office.

I'd always had an interest in Medicine and had studied Medical books extensively so with the bit of knowledge I had, I noticed the vials of fluid on the doctor's desk had quite a pinkish tinge to them.

Trying to act 'dumb', I asked the doctor what color a normal fluid should look like? He replied that it should be a very pale to creamy yellow.

I asked, "What if it isn't?"

He replied, "You see the vials, don't you?"

I said, "Yes."

Answering back, he said we shouldn't rush to worry as maybe he hit a vein, so he would send it to the Lab and let them tell us, but if it is blood from the fluid, we have a problem; but we'd just have to see what's there.

We went home and I was much more concerned than I let on to Larry.

I didn't want to alarm him in case he hadn't the same misgivings and feelings that I did. This was happening to him, not to me.

The doctor called shortly after and said he was going to rush the tests through and it would be a couple of days.

The next day, the doctor called and said the fluid showed there were Cancer cells throughout his entire body and all of his organs as well as his bloodstream.

The news came on January 4, 2000 and we had some decisions to make at that time.

We opted to come back and talk to the doctor and get a referral.

So, we did that. We were asked to go to the Cancer Center and talk to them to see what treatment they prescribed; whether it be Chemotherapy, Radiation or Surgery.

Larry was then sent back for another chest x-ray and from the time of the 1st one in December to this one in January, a larger mass had developed in the lung. His left lung.

The doctor had told us that he had planned to schedule surgery on the 21st of January. He was going to remove part, if not a significant part of the left lung.

I had been doing some research and knew that there were parts of a lobe of the lung that could be donated and I was willing to donate a section of my own lung for Larry if that would indeed help him.

Two days before surgery, the doctor called and said Larry's Cancer had advanced so rapidly that there is no need for surgery; they could not do anything as it had spread so far and it was encroaching upon his heart and around his Esophagus.

The tumor was over baseball size.

So after making an appointment, we went to the Cancer Center and talked to the Specialist there; the "Head Honcho".

They would talk to us about Chemotherapy and the side effects that would happen. Basically we wanted Larry to have Quality of life.

At this place in his diagnosis, nothing really pointed to Quantity, so we were into as much Quality as he could get.

We knew the surgery was out of the question and the doctors said they could go straight Chemo but no Radiation because the tumor had wrapped around his heart now and Radiation would destroy his heart.

We asked the pros and cons and spent a great deal of time discussing it.

What benefits could we expect? What could we expect at the end?

Would he be totally confined in the Hospital?

Once you start Chemo, can you stop? How long does it take to find out if it's helping? What is the expected outcome? What is the bottom line?

Armed with the additional research I'd done, I knew Chemo was NOT a cure!

At best, it would alleviate some symptoms and prolong things; and basically buy time, but I wanted to know how much time and if it indeed was going to be beneficial.

Larry hated above all thing, going to Doctors; tests; shots and needles; medicines; waiting, as well as going back and forth for an indefinite period of time.

I didn't want to have him go through all that if at the end, there wasn't any benefit for him.

The doctors were very sincere and honest with us and then they talked among themselves. After discussing all the options, reviewing all the records, examining Larry and understanding where the Cancer was and what it was as well as how fast it was progressing; one of the doctors replied, "I haven't seen anything progress this fast except a runaway freight train!"

We opted NOT to have Chemotherapy. We would do nothing.

This decision was because the doctors had told us in the final analysis, that at best, all they could venture to offer would be an extra month excluding all the side effects. Also, once begun, the Chemo could not be stopped. And, the quality would be gone. He would end up with a life without normality.

Cancer made it not normal!

Larry and I always decided that things would be as normal as we could possibly have it. We knew he'd be more comfortable and safe, being home and that's what he wanted. To stay home. He wanted to be around family, familiar surroundings and that was our plan. We knew that our relationship with each other was something that was so close; we were inseperable.

Yet, we felt better able to cope, the two of us, in our own private situation without making it a public issue.

We mustered all the postitive attitude we could and looked for the best answers. With the Lord guiding and directing our lives, whatever happens will be the Lord's will.

We aren't however just going to sit complacently by and do nothing.

The quantity is not nearly as important as the quality.

Larry had already had a Quadruple heart by-pass 13 years previous and we had the gift of those 13 precious years that otherwise we wouldn't have had. And that was a quality I would never exchange. I wasn't willing to have Larry be subjected to the Chemo and its prescribed horrors after what he'd already come through. The pain in Larry's chest, we thought was due to his heart, but it proved to be the Cancer.

*Understand this was not MY decision for Larry. We came to it together.

I am just sharing my thoughts through this ordeal from my perspective.

We knew the Cancer was going to change the family dynamics.

We have 3 grown children and 7 small grandchildren that were going to have to know about this but we wanted other people, really not to know anything more than; they're doing tests and we don't know 'exactly' what is going on. Yes, there's a problem. Larry has a paralyzed vocal cord, and try to leave it at that, without giving them the big "C" word. (Cancer)

For some reason, our society has an understanding that, if you have a cold, flu or pneumonia, you are treated normally; but, oh my goodness, mention cancer and they look at you and it's the "AWWWW" syndrome; the pity. "Oh, I'm so sorry."

I understand what they're saying but pity is something a Cancer patient; any patient doesn't want to hear. They want normalacy, they don't want this big "C" tattood on their forehead for the world to see.

They have to live with their diagnosis every day, so they don't want it pointed out to them and made the focal point of their life.

Larry and I had talked very deeply and we've always been able to talk about anything. We were trying to prepare for the changes that were going to take place and ask questions and get as much information as possible from anybody; doctors, nurses, research material too. I'd go to the library, talk to other people and listen very carefully.

Larry wanted to stay at home and not go to a hospital. The doctor had given him medication and said that as time went on, the pain would increase and the medication would have to be re-adjusted from time to time. We were to stay in touch and we did. We found out that our Insurance was inadequate and that we were not elegible for some of the services we needed and it would be a pre-pay situation on our behalf.

They would pay for us to see the doctor but as far as the medications, they weren't covered because Larry had to have the Name Brand and not the Generic. They just weren't sufficient in handling his pain; and of course, our HMO didn't cover that, so there were large amounts of money; hundreds of dollars per week.

It started out that Larry was on a small dosage, 3 mg. of Morphine, which very soon became inadequate to handle the pain.

In a very short time we drifted to 50mg. every hour, 24 hours a day. So, you can see that a prescription of 100 tablets costing over $100, was gone in a matter of 4 days.

Along with the expense of the medications, and his pain; Larry wasn't eating adequately. You know a Cancer patient must try to maintain as much weight, health, stamina and strength as they can, to fight the disease.

He was given a Steroid to increase appetite; the pain pill; anti-reflux meds; something to relieve nausea; another for Hives caused by yet another medicine.

On and on it would go. Pills, pills and more pills.

One bottle turned into two, then three, then five and so on.

I was then carrying a complete cosmetic bag in my purse, full of nothing but Larry's medicines.

One for appetite--moderate pain---extensive pain---etc.
My purse became bigger and bigger as his medicine bottles increases in number.

Larry and I had one super serious talk.
We were returning home from a doctor visit and we stopped at a church we had previously been to, for a Concert.
We remembered it had a pretty garden with benches where you could sit and talk. We wanted someplace away from everybody because there were important things we had to discuss.
We pulled onto church grounds and walked around a bit. They had been doing some new landscaping and the benches we had remembered, were gone; but there was a stair-step wall that we went and sat on, talking to each other; looking at each other and holding each other.
We cried and discussed how things were going to change our entire life.
We discussed how to tell our children that the Cancer would possibly take their fathers life; what he wanted me to do and what he wanted done; how he wanted to be treated.
Larry asked me one thing that's still pretty hard to talk about.
He asked that I be strong for him when he knew he couldn't be strong for himself.
Larry was always my strength, always there to support me and make me feel safe, and now I was to take that role, be his strength and make him feel safe. Whatever he needed; whatever he wanted, his life literally depended upon me and that's the way we both wanted it.
It was never an inconvenience or imposition to take care of Larry.
It was my absolute honor and privilege to take care of my best friend; the man I love more than my own life.

Larry told me that he knew from time to time, he would become very irritable and I was to understand that it was not him; and I shouldn't take it personal, for it was the disease.

You know that people who are ill are not always in the best frame of mind and they are not the ones to blame for this. It's the pain that makes this happen. I knew that and I resolved that no matter what he wanted, I would do my best to supply it.

I would run interference, so to speak, and muster up every ounce of strength I had, to keep things as normal as possible.

This was our "serious day" of discussion and I vowed after this, I would never let him see me cry. If I had emotions well up on me very quickly, I'd run through the kitchen to see if I had an onion to peel or maybe a sad movie that I could blame it on.

I had to keep "that look" off my face.

The 'look' of special concern, pity, or sympathizing because of what was happening before us.

I guess there comes an inner strength that each of us possesses; that God gave us to draw on at the opportune time.

I'm not saying it was easy because, Lord knows how hard it was; and to this day, how hard it is to hold all of your emotions perfectly calm within yourself and only supply the specific needs to your loved one; to be there; to fix an impromptu meal at the spur of the moment because immediately, his hunger could pass and he wouldn't have hunger again for a long while.

Larry could have given into a whim and become very demanding but he never did that to me. If he had asked me to stand on my head, I would have twirled batons with my feet and done anything to make him more comfortable, because he was the one going through this. I was on the sidelines. I was sharing it with him but I did not; and could not feel what he was feeling and I knew he was scared.

He always used to say,

"I don't like it when people say I have Cancer." "That's claiming it and who in their right mind would want to claim it?" "I don't have Cancer; Cancer has me." That was his attitude. It was nothing he had done. It was beyond his control. It was this blasted cancer that had a hold of him.

He could physically feel changes within his body; he could feel it growing and advancing by the increase in pain and now the difficulty breathing. Eventually we had to get oxygen support and he would trail 75 ft. of tubing from one end of the house to the other.

At the beginning, he only needed it at night to sleep and if he exerted himself too much.

We were still able to go for breakfast each morning because that was the best time for him to have an appetite.

It was probably his best, if not only, meal of the whole day.

It was always the same. Scrambled eggs with diced ham; toast and coffee.

Sometime later, it may only be a Sweetroll, but he would try to eat as much as he could because he knew it would be the best meal he would have that day and he had to have the calories.

Even though he had to take pills to increase his appetite, it would take a long time to develop that appetite each day.

If he wanted a milkshake, I'd give him a milkshake but I'd add an egg for extra Protein; extra Ice Cream for extra calories.

He didn't like the taste of those Nutritional Supplements. They were too sweet for him and just not satisfying.

He had one time, when he asked for: 3 chocolate donuts (cake, not glazed) with chocolate frosting.

I didn't care if it wasn't particularly healthy, if that was what he had an appetite to eat. Getting food into him and being able to maintain reasonable weight was more important than health.

He didn't have health anyway. The cancer stole that.

Before I forget----Hospice isn't always a choice or an end, but Hospice is available in its concept of care. I always thought of it as a building; to me, Hospice was a place. It is, but it's also a program and a way of thinking. These people are basically volunteers who provide spiritual and psychological support to terminally ill patients and their family. It stresses the quality of life, the peace, the comfort and the dignity. Their aim is to control pain and other symptoms so that the patient can stay as alert and as comfortable as possible.

The Hospice has nursing personnel also; which is key.

It becomes available and necessary when a person who wants to stay home, no longer can remain there because the benefit and treatment is no longer there. The Hospice can maintain support medically, psychologically and every way for the families; and the patient themselves.

The typical Hospice patient, when they enter, you hear they have a life expectancy of 6 months or less; that may be true but I found the "true Hospice" admission takes people who may have a week to 10 days left in their life cycle. This program tries to provide service in an atmosphere where the facility is to remain as comfortable as possible.

Hospice nurses have been through this transition. Every day they go to work and there is an end of life issue to be dealt with almost nightly.

These nurses also provide you with information and emotional support in facing this outcome and letting you know, you have done the right thing in choosing Hospice at this point.

Because of the care, it is more advantageous for the patient to get the kind of treatment they require, on demand and on a regular schedule; than to be at home helpless or alone and have to wait, sometimes through incredible pain for it to be controlled.

There is just so much, that can be done at home; and although it's a comfortable setting, I feel it should be left to the patient to decide whether to go to Hospice or not.

In our case, Larry did choose, at the end, because it became apparent that he could no longer be treated by the medication at home sufficiently.

He was taking medication but because he was no longer eating, he wasn't able to keep the medicine down. This being the case, the pain would get out of control and then, of course, because he couldn't eat, the medicine would make him violently sick.

There were times I would help him to the bathroom and he would lay on the floor knowing if he went back to bed, he would just find himself getting sick again, so he thought, "Why bother?"

I'm telling this like it is a Horror story because that's what it is; but you need knowledge in anticipation of what is happening and likely to transpire.

Let me walk you through a couple of phases that Hospice provided me with; things I could look for and be aware of, so things didn't come as a total surprise.

There is an actual breakdown and you know how to care for the person when you know what's coming.

A person approaches the end of their life in their own way and Larry chose to be private about it; to keep things as normal as possible.

People, not knowing there was anything really wrong, would treat him normal, because he looked physically well on the outside.

Let's face it; if someone knows you have a disability, physical degeneration or a terminal illness, you are definitely going to be treated different.

Though they'd say they would treat you normal, generally that is not the case. However we did find some of our very closest friends, and our Pastor, whom we shared with, did treat him normal; continued to tease him and treat him the way they always had.

They gave him the usual "hard time" and no pity.

I asked Larry at one point, "What do you want me to do with the rest of my life?"

He very briefly asked me to do three things.

1. "I want you to continue to write, because God gave you that gift."

2. "Paint because you enjoy it and it gives you peace."

3. "I want you to tell people how to treat a terminally ill patient as normal as you have treated me."

That is what I have tried to do.

Those that are going through the process that I have just come through.

I told you that Larry was diagnosed on January 4, 2000 and died on May 30,2000, in Hospice.

Hospice gives you a guideline of flexibility because what may happen in one case, may not present itself in another.

For some people it would take months to separate from their physical body and others may take only minutes. Death comes in its own time and its own way. It is as unique to the individual who is experiencing it, as snowflakes. There are no two cases exactly alike.

To try and put things on a timetable, I guess what I would have to say is; the most imminent changes start between one and three months before death actually occurs. The actual dying process begins about 2 weeks prior to death. There is a definite shift and change that occurs which takes the person from a mental processing of death to a reality comprehension, that their own mortality is coming to an end.

Unfortunately that understanding is not usually shared with others.

You have your first inclination that your knowledge says; yes you are dying and and it becomes real. Whatever you're dealing with inside, is kept private because you're trying to maintain everything in a normal way.

Larry never complained though you could see the pain in his face and he would ask for his pills but not make a big deal of it.

He'd just hold out his hand and tell me whether he needed an appetite or pain pill.

Slowly the person begins to actually withdraw from the world around them. They only feel comfortable with the people who are treating them as if nothing were wrong. They really don't like public displays or people dropping in, just to chat. No longer is that socialization important. They also begin to retreat from interest in newspapers; maybe television and finally their own family and children.

These people they love the most; because they don't want them to see the deterioration of themselves. They want everyone to remember them the way they were. They are, at this time, withdrawing from everything outside of themselves and going inside themselves. That is important because they are sorting out things that need to be done but inside yourself, there is only room for one.

That's yourself! Your life has to be put into perspective; there are things to do; there are things; if you have the time and knowledge, to make final plans for, in advance.

A lot of times, Larry could be seen processing things; whether it be pretending to be asleep or just quiet, so no one was particularly aware of what his thoughts were.

At a point, Larry decided he wanted to let the people that had been closest in his life, know how special they were to him; for he knew how blessed he had been by all of them.

Knowing in advance we had this time, he began making plans.

Sometimes people are taken so suddenly, that there is no time to make plans. He felt very blessed for this time.

In the midst of it all, Larry could only see blessings and more blessings.

He used to ask, "How many more blessings can I stand?" "I've been blessed more than anyone deserves to be blessed and I don't think I can hold any more." Then yet another blessing would come along, through an unexpected area; through the mail, a note, a neighbor, a card from the most unexpected places.

Also during this time, there is less need to talk. Words are a great part of the physical life and they tend to lose importance; but touch and smiles seem to compensate.

Eating tends to be a normal thing that slows down and finally ceases.

It is one of the hardest concepts for family and/or caregivers to accept because you consciously know they need the food and its energy for strength, but they just don't feel like eating. They have cravings though, that come and go. But, nothing tastes good. If they want it, whether you think it tastes good or not, give it to them. If they can, they will try to eat, but to deprive them of a craving; telling them they won't like it, serves no purpose.

Meats are probably the first thing to go because it is the most difficult to eat and digest, though it may taste good, it's very hard on the system.

Next would be vegetables and fruits until we're down to soft foods, like baby food and finally liquids. At this stage, it's okay not to eat.

There is a different kind of energy needed now. It isn't a physical energy anymore, it's a spiritual energy. You have one foot in each world.

One on Earth and one in Heaven, dealing with things, where food is no longer necessary. There seems also to be disorientation that goes on.

Sleeping seems to occupy most of the day. They can't seem to keep their eyes open. It's almost like they feel drugged but it's not from any medication. They're still able to be awakened from their sleep but it's the transition of having one foot in each world.

The person becomes confused about places and events, and you may even see them, at times, look right past you at someone or something you can't see. It may be a friend or loved one who had previously died and only visible to them.

There may be pulling or jerking of the bedclothes; arm movement resembling a tremor or agitation but without any purpose of physical activity that is grounding them to this earth.

They are no longer being grounded and are literally in the process of leaving. These motions might well be their way of trying to grab onto something for fear of drifting away.

Their blood pressure often lowers and there are changes in the pulse and the body temperature. For some reason which still puzzles me, their temperature vascillates between fever and chills. They're hot one minute and cold the next.

Even though there were times Larry ran a fever, there were other times he wanted the fan or air conditioner blowing directly on him.

There were times he had both fever and chills. Fever, but cold to the touch but he'd say he was hot. The body temperature fluctuated a lot at this point. Perspiration and clamminess with a skin color almost blue, on the bottom of his feet, while most of his skin was a pale yellowish pallor.

His nailbeds and his hands and feet were pale, as the heart cannot circulate the blood through the body with a normal flow anymore.

We didn't expect the time immediately after the diagnosis to be so short.

We asked the doctor what the chances were and he said that without further treatment, he'd probably have one to three months left.

We thought that wasn't quite optimistic enough so we asked another doctor.

He said that Larry had been strong and in good physical condition previously, so he thought Larry had from six to nine months.

That was still a short time but we thought we had some time to work;

The Lord had some time to work and we weren't going to panic here.

Though the time was limited, we chose to face it with optimism though it probably wouldn't change the outcome; we would face it in as positive a manner as possible.

It could definitely change the mood and the type of quality that was left for him.

We were prepared to accept whatever came next and we would live just one day at a time and be grateful for the time we had each day, with each other, and make it count for something.

Not everyone has time of any kind, as some are taken so swiftly, it almost seems like they were gone between heartbeats.

During the time after diagnosis, there was a period of coughing.

A suppressed cough, similar to a "tickle" in the throat but you couldn't clear your throat and sometimes it led to coughing up blood.

Now that I look back, I remember this happening on occasion and is one of the things that led us to the doctor, for which we were grateful.

Had this not occurred, there was a good possibility that we could have waited to see if the Laryngitis thing cleared on its own, which would have led to a much later diagnosis and resulted in no length of quality time. Larry told me, "If this is going to get me, then I'm going to get something out of it."

He wanted to go to Bora Bora but when I inquired, they told me of the long flight, transfers, handling our own baggage; all of which he couldn't physically handle.

I instead, looked into booking a cruise to Hawaii. We had never been on a cruise or to Hawaii. This would be stationary housing with all the amenities close at hand.

I knew what he was doing. He wanted me to have the pictures and memories, so in the future I would have it all to look back on.

He mustered up all the strength he could, to take this trip; for me!

Because he was worried about me. He wasn't worried about himself in the slightest; it was always me that he worried about. He was going to be alright. He was in a "win win" situation. It didn't matter to him.

No one comes into this life and leaves it alive anyway; and having known the Lord, he knew where he was going and the choice of staying here with the cancer or going to Heaven and walking with his Lord beside the Crystal Sea, was not even a choice.

If he were healed, that would be wonderful but if he went Home to be with the Lord, that was wonderful too.

He never looked at it as anything but a "win win" situation.

He felt sad indeed, for us that were left behind to still go through whatever our finality was going to be.

There were daily highs and lows which were very normal and there are the fears which are also normal.

Sharing time with me and our children, he was always ready to do for them whatever he could do to show them that things could still be normal.

His mental attitude was not outwardly consumed with his illness.

There was a sense of well-being about his future and knowing God was in control and regardless of what was happening, he was going to Praise the Lord.

We knew that each day was a gift and we were grateful for each and every one because before long, time would run out.

I'm writing this because #1, my husband asked me to keep writing and though I'm sure this wasn't exactly what he had in mind, it has become a joy.

I was asked by a man, to tell what I had been through because a relative of his was now going through the same thing and he felt completely helpless as what to say to her.

I couldn't seem to get to this point but somehow, putting it down on paper made it more real. It is a story that had to be told because there are people who can be helped from this, and if they can be helped to maintain any level of normalcy for the person they are giving care to, then it must be told.

To be in this position is a total aloneness; a total helplessness and a total hopelessness.

To stay normal within this, will require an abundance of courage, effort and strength. It's easier knowing that because of your great love for this person; giving and doing what you can, is the best gift you could ever give them and that is by giving of yourself.

Larry had decided that since his future was questionable, he wanted control of the things he had been collecting and who was to get them.

Our three children were called and asked to come for our 36th wedding anniversary on February 10, 2000.

Larry used so much of his energy in the next 3 days, sorting and boxing up everything he owned, to divide with the children those things that each would get.

Though I knew this could wait, I also understood how important it was for him to have "hands on" and the control when everything else in his life was out of his control.

He started the process of dividing things up. WE would roll dice, guess numbers like a private lottery, to decide who gets what, so there was no favoritism. It would be the "luck of the draw", so to speak.

He was a great collector of Toys and Tools.

There were Tonkas, Ertyl and Hot Wheels. All kinds of wonderful cars, trucks and tractors, most in original packages.

Larry was the boy who never grew up.

He didn't have toys as a child; he acquired them as an adult and now he was sharing his lifelong collection.

He also collected tools, mostly old primitive hand tools. Tools that were one of a kind that showed the quality workmanship that went into their making. He had been a "rough frame" carpenter and built homes.

So, tools were as much a part of him as the toys became. They were Larry!

He went to every Garage and Estate Sale he could find; picked them up at Auctions. He'd say, "Look, I found a tool I don't have."

He'd run to the local stores and get all the latest Hot Wheels to complete a Series and he treated them like a special Christmas present.

He'd say, "Oh, I found it." "This one was so hard to find."

Once he had a set completed, he'd start on another set. Always searching, always collecting, and now with great internal remorse, he was having to give them away.

He said to me once, "Now what am I going to do?" "There's no reason to go through the stores." "Nothing more to collect." But the curiosity was still there and we'd find ourselves at the store again discovering yet another new series.

He didn't stop. He never stopped. He never gave up! It became his private struggle to survive daily.

Through the countless hours of worry; rivers of tears and seeing the significant changes in his body, every day there was more deterioration.

Everyday through his love and zest for life, we maintained our wonderful relationship with each other and our children. Larry's faith was kept strong; joy of life prioritized. He wanted to find something that would take a really long time to do, so he would have that interest to keep looking forward to.

In February, for our anniversary, I asked the kids to come from their homes, to ours.

Our eldest daughter was in Alabama; our son was near Phoenix, Arizona and our youngest daughter lived in a nearby town at that time.

I wanted to get everyone together to have a family picture taken while their dad still felt and looked fairly good.

It had been 20 years since the last family picture because everyone had their own lives and agendas.

I also asked them to do some "homework". I knew I was always asking just one more thing of the kids, but I knew this to be of utmost importance.

What their dad was going through, he needed to know what his life has meant to the kids, and I wanted them to write letters to him and tell him what he's meant; what he's done and what it meant having him in their life.

Then I wanted them to read and share them with him.

A person who achieves something needs to be acknowledged for it and Larry definitely was not going to be denied that.

I knew each child may have difficulty.

It would take time and we'd stop whenever necessary to read them; talk about it; laugh and cry about it; whatever we needed to do.

But it would be something they could share; also be cathartic for them; something they needed to do, working through this.

They needed to adrenalize their feelings, their love and everything their dad had been and still was, to them.

It had to be put into words and Larry needed to hear this.

I had recently heard him say that it would be better if he died soon so he would no longer be in anyones way.

He needed to know how special he was and that he wasn't someone who would easily be forgotten. Because to know Larry, you could never forget him.

I even wrote and journalized what he meant to me, in my life with him; the years we'd shared together and everything we had done.

We set out that day with the appointment with the photographer.

We had the family photo taken with various poses. It was a lot of fun with the interaction. With the kids all here, it put an upbeat feel to everything.

Larry was upbeat and feeling well enough to participate in everything.

There was going to soon be a time when he wouldn't any longer want the kids around. It was an effort he had particularly made for them and this day. It was one more thing he had to put into place and perspective.

One more chapter in his "lifebook", in his preparedness to get ready for the end.

The everyday routine continued, so basically whatever he could do, we'd do.

Whatever he could not do, wasn't pointed out as his failure but rather an excuse by me, that maybe the weather wasn't going to be good or the sun was too hot; to justify a reason as to why our plans wouldn't be fulfilled. This way I hoped he wouldn't feel that it was because of his health.

Shortly after planning the reunion with the kids; waiting for the proofs to come back from the photographer, which couldn't happen fast enough, we questioned if we would run out of time? Would he feel like looking at the proofs? Would they be all that we had expected?

There was such a joy, the day the pictures came back and Larry was looking at them. There were pictures of he and I in back with the kids in front; he and I in front, with the kids in back; Larry and I alone with my arms around him, and a smile on his face of pure joy, as if to say he accomplished this and enjoyed it; and his kids are going to have a picture where he looked so good, rather than a sick old man.

It was very important to him that the kids not see him deteriorate before their eyes. They had already written, in their letters to him, what a strong example and hero he was to them; that it would have devastated him to see a look in their eyes that he was anything less than their hero, at this time of their life.

Larry wanted to go to Texas to visit his younger brother, Jon.

He had a special bond and relationship with Jon. They were the 2 younger of four children. His older brother and sister were quite a bit older and had already married when Larry and Jon were still kids at home.

A bond developed between them that in recent years they hadn't cultivated; and Larry knew he could count on Jon for keeping things normal.

[I know I use that work, normal, a lot but that was so important to Larry.]

Jon would do whatever he had to do, to make Larry comfortable.

There is no pretentiousness about Jon.

I called Jon to say we'd be flying to Texas.

Could he pick us up at the tiny airport near his home?

"No problem," he said.

So, we flew from Tucson to Dallas, changed planes to a small American Eagle and went into Longview. It was about 15 minutes from Jon's home and he was there to meet our plane. They were cordial and not overly affectionate because that would be too definitive that they might not get another chance to be together, but it was very normal!

Joking and kidding with, "Hey old man, want me to carry that suitcase for you?"

Just Jon's way of not having Larry feel incapable and catered to.

When we arrived at Jon's house, he showed us upstairs to the guest room.

He had put a small refrigerator there, in case Larry wanted water or Pepsi. He had run cable so Larry had Cable T.V. up there.

It had been over 20 years since Jon had made a CoffeeCake to share with his brother. He didn't just make one, he made three; in case Larry felt he could eat, Jon wanted there to be plenty.

Anything Larry wanted, Jon went out of his way. Not really out of the way, because that is just Jon and the way he is with everyone; only this recipient was his brother.

Munchies, the snack items; like chips; crackers & cheese; Reeses Peanut Butter cups; which were a real favorite of Larrys; had been packed and brought with us. The Cheetos; Crunch & Munch and anything chocolate.

He loved chocolate so much that locally on Sundays, after church, when we went to the Country Club for Buffet Brunch, even before Larry would have his salad, he would go to the dessert table to make sure he had something Chocolate for the end of his meal.

Once in a while he couldn't wait and before he was through with his salad, his chocolate dessert would already be gone and he justified it, as a reason to get more chocolate later in the meal.

Those were times when he was healthier.

Going to visit Jon was Family Time.

A diversion. Jon would keep things so interesting that Larry wouldn't have time to think about himself much. He was just enjoying being with his brother and his brothers' family.

Larry wanted to go to some Antique Malls one day and Jon said, "Okay, let's go."

We all got into the car and headed out. It wasn't too long; maybe 3 shops and that was it. Larry said he had to go back home and lie down.

"No problem," said Jon.

Not an inconvenience to him. Whatever Larry wanted.

"He's my brother", said Jon.

We'd go back to the house and Larry would sleep for awhile and I'd be downstairs talking to his brother and his wife.

Betty and I would fix dinner and see if Larry was hungry.

Sometimes he was and sometimes he'd just sleep through until morning.

There was one time that Larry slept 23 out of 24 hours, getting up only to go to the bathroom, get a quick drink and back to bed.

We made 4 trips in his last 6 weeks, all to see Jon.

It was like Larry couldn't get enough time together but couldn't ever say goodbye. Each time Larry was on Oxygen and since airlines wouldn't let anyone travel with full tanks of oxygen, for fear of explosion, this was a problem. People that need oxygen must carry empty tanks which renders the tanks totally useless. So Larry had to get permission from his doctor to be able to go without oxygen for a period of time during the flights.

The doctor said no, but Larry was determined to go; willing to suffer even if it killed him.

We decided to take with us, an Oxygen Capacitor, which was really a large suitcase with a motor that we'd plug-in and generate oxygen.

He had 75 feet of tubing to drag through Jon's house so he didn't have to carry the case. It was like being on a leash. He couldn't go any father than his tubing would allow.

After this last trip to Texas, Larry knew he'd never be back.

Jon did too, so when we left, Jon said, "Next time, we'll plan on Barbequing."

Larry answered, "Great, I'll bring the Watermelon from that fruitstand by the airport."

After arriving home and knowing there could be no more flying, Larry began getting depressed and wanting to plan the next thing he could get excited about.

He talked about a train trip across Canada or another Cruise.

I would go to the Travel Agent and obtain brochures to keep Larry interested and occupied. It worked. He had a lot to look over, fantasize about options he wanted, and during it all, I interjected comments about not being able to get prescriptions or medical assistance out of our area.

If something did happen out of Country, would I have a problem with extradition and getting him back home?

He heard my concerns as I knew he had, but neither of us ever actually said the words acknowledging the fact that further travel was impossible.

At this time, there were also some breathing changes, increasing to 70-80 breaths per minute and at times gasping for air.
When we had last traveled to Texas, Larry would take an extra pain pill, so he would sleep and his breathing wasn't so labored. There was some puffing and blowing of his lips when he slept, almost like he was blowing up a balloon, but he wasn't conscious of it and it never happened when he was awake.
We even thought of returning to Texas by car but the confinement and uncomfortable restraints, to say nothing of time to start and stop; made that impossible also.
His oxygen concentrater would have run off of its battery, as there was no place in the car to plug into direct current.
If we took oxygen in tanks, we would have to carry a lot, or stop to fill them quite frequently. It would almost sound more doable to travel by ambulance; what with all the paraphernalia that we would have to take with us.

I decided that if he wanted to go back to see his brother, there wasn't anything I was going to do to stop him.
It was his life. It was his wish and if we spent 3 days driving to see Jon; 3 days visiting and 3 days returning home; at least he would have those 3 days with his brother, which he desperately wanted. So, I thought, what was I trying to protect him from? What would be so different?
He was ill and not going to get better whether or not he went or stayed.
What was better? Here, or being with his brother and having distractions?

29

Here, Larry was more isolated; going from room to room, sleeping, doing a jig-saw puzzle and feeling confined like a prisoner.

So I decided, for him I would relent and not try to talk him out of it anymore, because I had said from the beginning that whatever Larry wanted, I was going to do.

I was trying to be very protective and I understand now, that it bordered on pity, protection and sympathy; all the things he didn't want.

In order to maintain this normalcy--- "Sure, lets' go honey."
And we did go, one more time.

This was the final trip and one week after we returned, was most difficult for him. But, he had something that could never be taken away; another chance to see his brother and have their picture taken together.

I think it was the best medicine because he had happiness.

Though they both knew this was the final goodbye, nothing was said about it aloud though at the airport, there was a special hug.

There was the same comment, "See you next month."

This time Jon had no way of knowing that when he said that, it would be Jon coming here the next month for Larry's Memorial Service.

Surprisingly, Jon was the only one from Larry's immediate family that came. That would have really hurt Larry, so it was just a blessing that he never knew about it.

The service was videotaped and Larry planned the message to be one of Salvation as his family wasn't saved. This was his intent, that his siblings could come to know the Lord, as he had.

Larry deteriorated rapidly after this last trip. In a matter of 2 days, his breathing pattern became much slower. He depended upon his oxygen 24 hrs. a day and he was on a level of 4 liters.

It didn't however, seem to ever be enough.

Walking to the bathroom was almost too much exertion and the 2nd day back, he didn't bother getting dressed anymore.

He stayed in his pajamas and basically stayed in bed. Everything became enhanced. Sounds and smells. I could no longer cook food because the smell made him sick. Candles; any candles that were in the house had to be removed even if they were never lit. The smell was overwhelming to him.

Even to the point that the canulla that went into his nose from the plastic oxygen tubing, bothered him; so much that I would sit in bed with my back against the wall with Larry sitting between my legs, leaning against my chest. I would hold the canulla in front of his nose so he could get oxygen and let him sleep that way.

I could only do this for periods of 2-3 hours at a time because my arms would go to sleep and I'd have to change positions so I did have to keep moving him or having him move; and this is where his sleep deprivation came in.

I knew the pain was greater; his sense of smell, more intense; his agitation also was growing.

Everything was coming to a total intense restlessness, which I knew was due to an increasing lack of oxygen in the blood and brain.

I could see that his skin was looking wax-like, that yellowish tone.

His nails were blue as were his feet. In fact they looked like someone had used a stamp pad to get footprints.

He was cold to the touch, all the time. But he had to have the air conditioner on. It felt almost like a refrigerator in the house but Larry said it was easier to breathe if it was cold.

When our daughter would visit, she would wrap up in a blanket and say, "I feel like a Burrito," She would just shiver. I guess I got used to it, though at times I'd put on a sweater. I tried to keep Larry's body temperature up, by keeping our bodies close in bed.

I've always thrown off a lot of body heat but it soon became difficult sleeping in the same bed because he was becoming so sensitive to touch and movement. The sheets touching his skin would hurt. He was restless because he couldn't lie down. On his back and side; he couldn't breathe.

Even in a recliner, he couldn't get comfortable. His legs would dance. There was just such an anxiousness in every movement he made.

I tried to keep him hydrated with juices. He would drink grapefruit juice, orange juice and chocolate milk with a straw. He could no longer drink from a glass without the straw because he would choke. He said the liquids were too thin. Some juices were better because of the consistency but soon everything began to make him choke. Whatever he wanted to try, I'd supply.

The second day back from Texas was also eventful because Larry's oral pain medication was no longer effective and I had to call the doctor stating I thought we were getting to the point of having to have injections because nothing I have here, at home, is effective anymore. That's when the doctor told me he would contact a Home Health Nurse to come out with Morphine Suppositories to see if he could be stabilized that way.

She did come and stayed for a couple of hours going over instructions for me. She said she would come back one more time but wasn't usually allowed to return twice in the same day. But, because the pain could not be abated, I had to keep calling for more and more refills. I became his nurse and administered all the suppositories. I bathed him in bed as he didn't leave the bed anymore. There also developed no urgencies for body eliminations anymore.

He would go days at a time without going to the bathroom and that concerned me because I knew that meant the body was shutting down.

I again called the doctor and said that I didn't know what else to do. We had talked about putting a Hospital bed in the Living Room but we were coming upon the Memorial Day weekend and there were a lot of things we couldn't obtain because of the Holiday. There was paperwork to be taken care of to reserve the equipment. It was a terrific effort to arrange in a timely manner. The doctor was phenomenal in pushing everything through and it finally came down to the fact that nothing more, pain wise, could be handled at home and that is when I told Larry that I didn't think I could maintain his comfort anymore. They needed to get him stabilized somewhere and then come back home where he would then be receiving injectible Morphine.

That was the plan we were anticipating.

Larry didn't want an IV set-up. The doctor was concerned about that but Larry said no. He didn't want anything invasive.

He had signed a Living Will and stated he didn't want to be artificially maintained. No heroics or resuscitation.

He didn't want to go to a hospital if at all possible; and those were his words, "No hospital if at all possible."

And now, I was beginning to feel that I was abandoning what we had agreed on, as far as his wanting to stay home; so I was letting him down because my only alternative was to send him to Hospice where people could manage his pain 24 hrs. a day.

He and I were both exhausted. I hadn't left the house. I couldn't even go to our mailbox because something could happen and so I just stayed inside.

Neighbors would call and I would ask if they could bring the mail to the house because I couldn't go out. I couldn't go to the grocery store or anywhere. I was actually confined to the house with Larry, afraid to leave.

I had neighbors who had offered to come in and just sit with him but I knew he didn't want that because they were 'outsiders'; so I stayed.

There were things in the freezer we hadn't used; I couldn't cook because of food odors and he wasn't eating anyway so whatever we had, was out of a can, jar or bottle. I had juices and milk in the house. We weren't going to starve. We could live quite a while on the amount he was able to consume; in fact now his intake was completely liquid. I told Larry the only way to maintain his pain was to go to a hospital and he surprised me by saying, "Yes."

When I called the doctor, he said it would take a little while to arrange things and he'd get back to me. The 'little while' took 6 hours and it was way into the evening, about 9 PM when the word came through that he was approved to be admitted to Hospice.

We are now arriving at Hospice. Larry was transported by ambulance. He was by himself, staring out the backdoor windows. He didn't request that I ride with him. I believe he realized this ride, he had to do alone.

I drove myself, and arrived at Hospice just as they were settling Larry into bed and hooking up oxygen.

The first night, I came home; thinking he would get a better nights' sleep if not worrying about me. He did.

So, I went home again the 2nd night.

I received a phone call from Hospice about 5AM. The nurse told me that Larry had become quite agitated and restless in the night. I answered, "Yes, I told you that between 2AM-6AM were his worst times of agitation and you had it documented."

She said, "Well, we didn't have anyone in the room, and he fell out of bed, bruising his face and shoulder badly."

He had fallen face first onto the floor and I said, "That's it; I'm coming in right now."

From that point on, I never left Hospice again. I never left his side. I slept in a chair beside his bed and never left him for the next 5 days. I bathed there, changed clothes there. I ate there. My daughter joined me and brought clothes and food because I wouldn't leave the room. I stayed, and talked to him as if he

34

could coherently understand me. Dawn (daughter) brought my CD player from home to softly play his favorite music. We put it under the bed so it wouldn't be too loud. I would also read to him. I kept a journal continuously and he was very restless and was always saying he wanted to go home.

The doctor and I both had said, "Larry, you have to wait until after Memorial Day weekend is over because we can't arrange anything sooner."

I said, "Honey, you just have to wait until Tuesday." [that was the day after Memorial Day]

Larry just looked at me so sad and said, "I won't be here then."

I knew what he meant, but I was hoping that maybe one more time he'd be able to go home.

He didn't much like hospitals but I think he knew this time he had to resign himself to endure this because it was a burden off me and he knew no one could take further care of him at home adequately, even though he wanted to be home.

Hospice was a mixed metaphor for me. On one hand I thought I had let Larry down. I had done my best on what we had agreed to; keeping him at home and private, so now I had somehow come to fail him.

Then I also thought I had failed our marriage vows;
in "sickness and in health," that I should be the one taking care of him.

But my capabilities had run out and I had a lot of torment with that, as well as a lot of discussions with the Hospice nurses who kept trying to reassure me that I had done the right thing.

I know now that I did do the right thing and the best thing for him; by getting him the best care and not just what was adequate with my limited skills.

He was safe. He was taken care of and comfortable in bed, while being monitored and kept pain free on a regular schedule.

This was the best I could do for him and I now know that. At the time, it didn't give me much peace.

His hands and feet were now becoming more splotchy and purple around the knees and down the shin area. His hands would stay in an almost fixed position; partially relaxed and open with his fingers gently bent. We would be constantly rubbing cream and oils on him to keep his skin soft and also keeping his lips moist. for the most part, he had completely quit taking anything by mouth, including water.

I asked him one afternoon if he wanted a drink of water and he shook his head yes, as it was almost impossible for him to speak anymore. He had lost that capacity. You had to put your head practically on his chest with your ear near his mouth, as he could barely make a whisper.

I turned to get a cup and when I turned back, Larry had taken the whole water pitcher form his tray table and was trying to drink from it, not realizing what he was doing. I gently took it from his hands and said, "Let me pour you a cup, honey."

Once again he whispered to me, "I'm not going home again, am I?"

I said, "We're going to try to get you home."

One of the nurses who had been standing in the doorway, left; and a few minutes later returned with a quilt in her hands. Thought we always had a fan gently blowing on Larry and he was sensitive to touch, we gently pulled up the sheet and put the lightweight quilt on top, not for warmth but for mental comfort. He could feel it with his hands on top of the covers. He opened his eyes wide, and although glassy, almost looked like he had tears in his eyes. he turned and looked toward me, whispering, "Honey, am I home?"

I said, "Yes honey, you're home."

I knew he was never going to leave here. After that, Larry became mostly unresponsive and unaware of his environment.

The next opportunity we had, we removed the quilt, folded it and put it on a shelf in the corner. He was no longer aware of the original existence of the quilt. It had done its job.

From time to time, Larry would make gestures that we didn't understand. That was yet another closure with one foot in this world and the other foot in another.

Sometimes he would raise his right arm like he was pointing or reaching for someone to take his hand and mouth something inaudible. He'd then shake his head affirmatively and then whisper, "Okay, okay."

He was obviously conversing with someone that was not visible to us and I'm sure it was probably his mother or someone else who had gone to the Lord already.

It was evident of the vast deterioration and within 4 days, his care was limited to turning; medication and bedbath. he could slightly be roused, but for the most part, had become unresponsive.

He did seem to be aware of my voice which indicated he was still here, but didn't open his eyes.

Dawn was there as frequent as possible, although in the process of moving from her apartment back home with me.

She'd talk to Larry, and told him she had to leave, as she had one more carload to get. She also said she'd be back by evening, as it was now 2PM.

She had no sooner gone, than Larry opened his eyes, crooked his finger gestering me closer to the bed. I put my head near his chest. He reached up with both arms and put them around me and drew me close. he whispered, "My life with you has been awesome." "I love you so much." and then kissed me.

Instantly he lapsed into a coma.

I think he was waiting for Dawn to leave so she wouldn't see him lapse.

He never woke up again.

Things happened intensely over the next 4 days. We basically talked to him, read to him, massaged his legs and feet, making him as comfortable as we could.

Nurses would come in to bathe him.

They would bathe from the waist up, while Dawn and I bathed from the waist down; this way finishing at the same time and as quickly and efficiently as possible.

One nurse made a comment about how Larry must be loving 4 women massaging him. He would have found humor in that statement. We placed his arms and hands on pillows to relieve pressure. His blood pressure would go up and down; his pulse increased and decreased; the color of his skin would change.

Even though we had sweaters on due to the fans, Larry would still sweat profusely.

He developed breathing that became very loud and I asked the nurse if it could be lessened by putting him on one side or another and she said yes; if he were on the side away from his heart, it would ease some but still come and go. This transition he was now making, was becoming more evident. He was moving away.

In hindsight I can see exactly when it started. It became present about a week earlier and now progressing faster and it continued so we just maintained and kept on keeping on.

Talking, combing his hair, stroking his hand, relieving pressure points kept things stable. His legs were extremely blothchy now.

At this last stage, in days or hours, things happened that don't manifest in everyone. The nurses were reluctant to elaborate because the various things that could happen, may not happen and even if you knew, you wouldn't be prepared for it.

His eyes were partially open so nurses would put cream in, so they wouldn't dry out.

Because he wasn't taking any fluids, we had to frequently swab his mouth with a moist sponge-stick and his first involuntary reaction was to tighten his lips like the swab was a sucker.

Then he wouldn't let go. He wasn't aware of it. It's something everyone does. There was no final surge of energy that we were told we might expect. There was a decreased urine output even with a catheter. He would have been devastated by that, so I'm grateful he didn't know he had a catheter.

There was an episode of his breathing that really alarmed me. It was like he had a bad cold and there was a raspiness in his throat.

He began to have fluid retention in various parts of his body. Under his chin, it became hard and swollen where fluids were settling. This swelling occurred within a half hour and it wasn't something we were prepared for. It was actually like a huge growth that had just developed and made his throat look like a quadruple chin.

His skin had a tendancy to bruise with blood vessels breaking and at that time, his skin looked paper thin. I was told that his ear lobes could turn black, in the last stages; as well as his hands and feet would become mottled purple.

I understood that was the bodys way of giving priority to the heart and brains inability to oxygenate properly.

The hearing is the last to go. I remember being told that in 1989, when my sister was dying of cancer.

The nurses told me to sit by his head and talk to him. It was necessary to tell him that it was okay to go; and that everyone would be alright; and I would take care of everything because if you grieve in front of them, they feel the stress of your grief and it's too much for them to process and delays their passing peacefully.

I remember my sister fighting and fighting until I was able to calmly reassure her that is okay to let go; we would miss her, but if she was seeing a light, that she should go toward it as fast as possible and not stay and delay the process because her release would set her free from the pain.

As I sat by Larrys head, I told him lovingly, the same thing.

"Honey, I know you worry about me all the time as I worry about you, but it's okay now because you only have one last mile to go; and if you've reached that mile, go quickly and peacefully because I'm going to be alright and I have given you back to God and He's going to take care of you now, because I can't."

"I loved you very much and I'll always love you."

I knew then, that everything would be alright.

Cancer is not discriminative of age or person.

With Larrys Lung Cancer, the symptoms of the Pulmonary function developed into coughing, which I was told happens to 75% of the patients. It's an agitated cough like you have a "tickle" rather than a cough resembling a cold. This is usually combined with blood because of the cough force. A third of patients exhibit shortness of breath, which I thought was extremely low. Also a quarter of patients have chest pain. Again, I'm surprised that number is so low. Larry had extreme chest pain.

His laryngitis didn't seem to be a fluke. Hoarseness is developed by 18% of people with Lung Cancer and a lot of time there is a paralysis of the diaphragm restricting breathing.

Larry would often say he couldn't get enough air to take a breath. I actually thought it was just shortness of breath but instead, it was his diaphragm so full of cancer preventing his air intake.

This wheezing or vibrating breathing almost sounded like Bronchitis or Asthma, but with fluid in it. It is a moveable, wet, congestion that had to be suctioned several times to keep from drowning in his own bodily fluids.

At one point, I counted his breaths and it reached upward to 140 times a minute, which would put any one of us into hyperventilation. At the same time, it was like Larry was gasping for air and still breathing like a race horse who had just run a race and was trying to catch his breath.

That was pretty hard to listen to and it's known as a "death rattle."

I had thought because of the name, there would be more of a "rattle" and there wasn't.

My daughter had just come by, bringing dinner, even though it was almost midnight.

She was exhausted, so I told her to curl up in a lounge chair and that I was going to journal, sitting by her dads bed.

She told me that I should get some sleep because I hadn't slept for almost 52 hours and was feeling shaky. But, I said no, because I was afraid if he started gurgling, I wouldn't hear him and if I weren't alert to suction him, he may choke. So, I stayed awake journaling, holding his hand, letting him know I was there.

Dawn was finally asleep and I was subconsciously listening to his breathing which was almost rhythmic because I was now used to it.

Suddenly, it change drastically. That is to say, it became normal and quiet. It was a normal breath but shocked me at the same time.

I jumped up, hit Dawn on the bottom of her feet and said, "Wake up, his breathing has changed." I ran around to the other side of the bed. She went to the side closest to her. I was stroking his hair, saying, "It's okay honey, it's okay."

The next breath also was a normal one but he had a period of apnea, about 15 seconds, and then another normal breath, which was his last breath, and he was gone.

I said to Dawn, "Dad's gone."

She looked at me and said, "Mom, he can't be."

And I said, "He is, honey."

I rang for the nurse and she came in with a stethoscope and listened. I looked at her without any imparted words, then asked, "Is he gone?" She cocked her head to one side, not acknowledging affirmative or negatively; then left the room.

I knew he was gone.

It was very peaceful; that last 20 seconds. [2:23AM]

I always knew that 2 in the morning was a very agitated time for him, and a time of great distress; to see him peaceful was unusual, but reassuring to me in a strange way.

So, Dawn being on one side of the bed and me on the other; we said our goodbyes. We stroked his hair; we kissed his forehead; held and kissed his hands and his cheek.

I told him how much I loved him. I told him how sad I was, not to be going with him; because that's the way I felt. It wasn't fair; he was going and I had to stay, without him. He was my "best friend in the world."

Then another nurse came in with a stethoscope, a Supervisor, and she listened. She said nothing and went out, closing the door behind her. I knew she was giving us time to say goodbye.

I knew that I could NOT stay there and watch them come in and take him from me. I had to leave. I told Dawn, "Let's get our stuff together and get out of here." "We need to go home."

"Dad's not here anymore." "Your dad's gone; gone home to be with the Lord."

Now, I hadn't slept for almost 60 hours and I still had a lot of things to do. We decided to stop and get a cup of coffee on the way home. We stopped at a local Circle K, and while I was driving, I was going over in my head, what Larry and I had talked about concerning the Memorial Service. I had added a few things because I wanted it to be special. My one last time to let "my Larry shine."

His private struggle was over. It was going to be public knowledge. It was no longer, 'private.'

He had helped me arrange what he wanted for his service.

He wanted everybody he knew, to know how much he loved them, so we had written little "one liners" about each of his friends and acquaintances, that were read at his service.

The doctor came to his service. He spoke and wept at the courage and the love of life that Larry had; and the lesson he had learned from Larry. To count all your Blessings and in everything--give God the Praise and Glory.

Larry never complained and I think he had so much to complain about. He was so concerned about sparing me or upsetting me, that he was the one who actually made everything remain normal; because there is nothing normal about this disease.

Every case is different. Some are easier than others. Some are much longer and tormenting than others.

Larry was diagnosed on January 4, 2000 and he died May 30, 2000.

He was 60 years of age. He was too young. I think the thing that bothers me the most in my grief and aloneness is; remembering that my husband, who loved life so much, is not here to enjoy it.

I will keep the promise that I made to him; I will continue to write.

Hopefully in some small way, I have been able to fulfill Larry's hope of telling how to treat someone with a terminal illness, as normally as he had been treated.

There were 12 rooms at Hospice and I donated 12 comforters, hoping others would be able to experience the peace Larry had found through the comforter placed on his bed.

I heard that family members were taking these comforters home as a last momento of a loved one. When I would bring new comforters to replace those taken, I suggested that a donation be made by those taking the comforters so they could be replaced in order to make sure every patient would continue to have one.

I wrote something for Larry's Memorial Service that I would like to end with.
As a tribute to Larry, I had this poem inscribed on a plaque and hung on a wall at Hospice. It has also been read at monthly Hospice Memorial Services.

The Comforter

A man lay still in a lonely bed
A pillow gently cradling his head
The sheets felt so harsh
For they were quite starched
No comfort could be found.
An understanding nurse went looking around
And a quilt she did find, with blue and red
She gently laid it across his bed.
The man touched the fabric and was instantly soothed
Not from warmth but comfort here;
It eased his mind, and calmed his fear.
Soon this man opened Heavens' door;
Stepped inside and was here no more.
Before he departed for Heavens' crest,
He turned and smiled, for he had been blessed.
May the comforters upon this bed; each one
Give you peace when day is done.
And know this too, without a doubt.
God also is a Comforter who will help you out.
Just reach out and touch Him, with your hand

And know His comfort will help you stand.
Strong, you will walk, that same Heavens' crest;
Knowing that The comforter has given you rest.

In memory of my husband:
Lawrence Richard Hoffman
"Larry"
December 11, 1939--May 30, 2000

"Larry, we hold you in our heart
God holds you in His hand."
Good Night!

Pain is inevitable. We can't prevent it, and sometimes we can't stop it once it's started. But we can choose not to be miserable.
Invite Jesus to come into your fiery furnace with you, and He will place His loving hands under you and lift you up into His strong arms of protection.

In your grief, go limp, and let others carry you for a while.
In doing so, you'll make a friend!

While we're not really sure where Heaven is, the Bible often refers to it as being up or above.
That produces one of the "side effects" of heavenly thinking. when we're focusing on the joy we'll know in Heaven, our thoughts turn heavenward---that's upward.
Our hopes rise, and life down here is more bearable.

Music has been a golden thread woven through the tapestry of my life, bringing joy into the dark areas.

Sharon J. Hoffman

Music reminds me that God's enduring love runs throughout my life and into eternity, a symbol of His promise that someday I'll be rejoining my loved ones in heaven to sing praises to our Lord in person.

One of the best bonuses about being---or just acting---joyful is that inevitably the joy we share is reflected back to us just when we need it most.

The blessings that come from reaching out to others cannot be overestimated.

Reminiscing helps us put our lives into perspective.
As we get older, we can see how each stage, every memory, fits into the grander scheme of things.
My life has included sorrow as well as happiness.
And all those emotions, all those bittersweet memories have created what I like to think of as a bright, colorful, firmly woven tapestry.

Somewhere I read that for every single thing that goes wrong in our lives, we have fifty to one hundred blessings.
What we need to do is learn to identify those blessings and spend more time counting---and being thankful for them!

Those who hope in the Lord will renew their strength.
They will soar on wings like eagles; they will run and not grow weary, they will walk and not be faint. Isaiah 40:31

Just imagine living where love fills our lives so completely there won't be any empty spaces left in us to fill. Therefore we won't want anything. We'll be perfectly content--supremely satisfied. And since that will surely be the case, it seems quite likely that our heavenly palaces won't need to be very big because we won't have any stuff to store.

It's not easy to be the one to survive.

I feel as if I'm in a "waiting place."

Not a waiting room but a place to wait.

Waiting to feel something besides

grief, loneliness, fear, sadness, depression, forgotten, alienated, abandoned, helpless, pitied, hopeless and did I mention, fear?

Fear of being alone, becoming ill, falling and not being found and even dying.

Maybe it is just an age thing, but before my husband died, I never gave daily or even frequent thoughts of my own mortality.

Everything I encountered before in my life, suddenly changed the minute I became a widow.

Time at that moment, had no importance or value as it had when I had someone in my life to share with.

I had no time schedule anymore for eating, sleeping, shopping, preparing meals, going home, being home or working.

In fact, motivation was in short supply and indifference became top of daily activities.

It seemed that time had suddenly expanded.

There was so much more of it un-scheduled as well as so much left to endure alone.

As you may have noticed, I mentioned having no schedule for being home or going home.

Being self-employed, I soon lost desire to continue working. I began to live on savings.

Eventually as time passed and finances dwindled, I was forced to step back into reality to survive; but I must admit, my interests had changed and I had to force myself into self-motivation.

Luckily I had the foresight to complete an advanced education which I now had to resort to, for future income.

sharon004d嗯

My life indeed took a 180 degree turn as I ventured into the new career of counseling those who were terminally ill as well as those who were just entering the world of loss and grief.
In helping others, I hoped to gleen more than I gave and that my healing would find a beginning.

Adjustments are a day to day event.
The list continues to grow and things I used to take for granted now have to be done differently and perceived differently in my head.

1. I went from being alone and single to having a partner and being a couple.
2. From caring for myself to caring for another.
3. Bearing children and sharing time and goals while cultivating mutual friendships both socially and in extended family.

I perceive life as jigsaw puzzles to complete and each milestone is another completed puzzle.
The day Larry died, it was to me, as if all the completed jigsaw puzzles in my life to that time had been separated and tossed into a bag where now it looked overwhelming to begin singling pieces from each separate phase of life and starting the task of sorting, salvaging and re-assembling each individual puzzle into a life for me---minus a "key" piece from each puzzle.
The end result will never be complete without that "key" piece, no matter how hard one tries.
Something will always be different and each time there is another loss or life change, more "key" pieces are removed until there is nothing any longer recognizable to piece together.
It is forever new and changing but never again able to be fully completed. the attempts are there but they always remain attempts.

Starting over again and again is stressful and each time it is more difficult and less motivating until it could be totally reasonable and understandable to put less and less effort, interest and energy into it any longer.

The inevitable may be to begin and end each day as a separate journey; always starting at ground zero and returning to ground zero at night.

I was once told that one should think of a game of golf as 18 separate games beginning and ending at each hole, instead of one game consisting of 18 holes, not completed until after the 18th.

That pretty much summed up the way I looked at my future without Larry.

It would be "one lifetime in a day", which would repeat 365 time and then repeat another 365 days--except for leap year--for the rest of the time that I remain alive.

I never thought about making plans past today because just getting through today seemed an immense task that I was no longer sure about.

There certainly wasn't as much motivation or reasoning to make decisions about the future when I had so much difficulty dealing with the present.

I question daily about when this empty feeling would end and I could begin to see improvement in my outlook for another beginning.

I promised my husband that I would not harm myself and I'd never broken a promise. I had tried never to make a promise because circumstances can nullify your intent; and though I would say, "I'd do my best", I would not make idle promises because I believe people should stand by their word and be judged that way.

Sharon J. Hoffman

Larry knew the depth of my love for him and why I was questioning as to how I'd survive without him here by my side, and that was the reason he asked for my promise. I thought about it, and though "I'd do my best", this wasn't sufficient for him and his peace of mind in having to leave me behind.

I also knew that if I made him a promise, I'd be life bound to keep it.

I did promise him what he wanted and I must confess---there have been times I've tried to figure out how to get around that promise.

In the last ten years, many times I've been so unhappy and sadly hopeless without him.

I reviewed the exact words of my promise.

I know I promised not to harm myself personally, (which meant taking my own life), but I never promised I wouldn't let life--take me.

I figured if I just stopped eating and drinking and lay down in bed, I'd eventually die in my sleep.

Theoretically that was well and good but I didn't count on my conscience or my memories to make me question my promise to Larry.

It took about 3 days to rationalize what I was doing. No matter how I tried to justify it, I knew I was in the throws of breaking my promise. To quit trying to live and just give up, was the same thing as breaking my promise not to harm myself.

I'd never be able to endure that betrayal.

You may ask, "How would Larry ever know?"

That didn't matter! I'd know!!

There are many things in my life I'd like to have done over or different or better; but, no way to ever reconcile my breaking a promise. Never! That's not the type of person I am, or who I raised my children to be, either.

I knew it was going to be terrible and I would have many moments, days and possibly forever to grieve, but it was the "hand I was dealt" and I'd stay in the game of life and play it out, the best I could.

People say that time heals all wounds..

I say it depends on the person and the wound.

For me, I am still trying to heal and after ten years, I have good and bad days. I have come a long way but I haven't finished the journey and may never accomplish the healing that people have talked about.

Maybe that saying was originally said, to give hope.

Maybe it was said, out of desperation or ignorance of the reality.

I don't say that I loved---deeper than anyone else because I believe love and feelings are so very personal.

I can say I loved my husband more than anyone else did.

Everyone has a different relationship and various degrees of love.

I couldn't love your husband, wife, brother, sister, son or daughter as you do.

And you can't know to what degree I loved my husband, either.

These are intimate and personal feelings known only unto ones self.

Healing also depends on personal faith and support. I had a very small support group.

My children were suffering as I was and though we grieved simultaneously, we were not independently strong enough to be of constant support to each other.

My pastor and a very few friends were all I had.

Most people didn't know how to help, so did nothing.

I admit that if anyone came to my home for a visit, I didn't open the door.

They never knew whether I was inside. They only knew no one answered the door. That was my own choice.

I didn't want kind words at that time.

I wanted my husband back and since that wasn't going to happen, I didn't want to hear what anyone had to say.

How could they possibly know what I was feeling? The loss and the despair were devastating to me.

After all, they would return home and be able to sit at the dinner table, watch T.V., talk and retire to their beds for the night with their spouse and family.

I was going to do the same---but alone.

Alone for the rest of my life!

There are those that are quick to tell me that in time, I will get over my grief and be back to normal. This is my normal!!!!

They say I might even date again and possibly re-marry and have a new life.

NOT!!!

I'll never get over----I may get through;--and just what is, 'back to normal?' That would be having Larry back!! That would be my 'normal.' And re-marriage----let me just say: "I don't judge or condemn those who think that way; but for me it is not ever going to happen.

I had spent over 36 years married to one man and sharing everything in life with that one man, who was also my best friend!

One I could laugh with; cry with; and share dreams as well as secrets with.

To begin again and replace all the memories of my past is unthinkable.

My children are grown and I have been an effective independent person.

I don't need another person to share an intimate relationship with--in my life.

I live alone but I am not lonely.

People are in my life because I want them there, not because I need them there.

If I desire companionship, I can go out for an evening or event.

But, at the end of the evening, I go home alone.

That also is my choice!!!

I choose to keep busy---maintain friendships, though different than when I was married.

I now can devote my unencumbered time, doing things with others; for others, and extract whatever healing I need for myself from each experience.

I totally understand others' needs or desires to begin another relationship and even get married again.

It is just that though,--a personal choice.

I too, have made my personal choice.

At my age, I want something to devote the rest of my life to, that will give me satisfaction and fulfillment without a personal intimate commitment.

It is still a personal involvement but one of service and not self-seeking of the heart.

I had that and it was wonderful.

I lost it and must move ahead in a different direction.

I chose further education and a chance to give something back to society.

Since my situation showed me that most people had little knowledge of grief and the whole process; and it was a subject few wanted to talk about, it was the perfect path for me to pursue.

Maybe by talking to others and sharing ideas and opinions, would not only give me insight in their feelings, but help me deal with my own feelings.

Sharon J. Hoffman

In the long run, I hoped to do, with the rest of my life--something both I could be happy with, and Larry would have been proud of me for!

"I still love him more than all the stars in the sky!!!!!!!!!!!!!!"

Tears In My Pocket

Each morning when I wake up and get out of bed, I am aware that it is another day alone.

No one to say 'Good Morning' to; no one to fix breakfast for; no one to include in the plans for the day.

Just one heart beating but the silence in the house is almost deafening.

No matter how much time goes on, I am not used to the utter silence surrounding me. The only noises I hear are house noises.

The furnace cycling on and off; the refrigerator doing the same; the ringing in my ears that I am now quite aware of.

Mostly the overwhelmingly 'loud' silence.

I spoke to a friend the other day who had lost her husband in late February.

She asked me, "Will it ever get better?"

I told her that it wouldn't necessarily get better but it would be different.

There seems to be a pattern in moments of grief.

There is the initial shock and disbelief before it becomes reality.

There are times of fond memories and times of utter hopelessness.

Each day brings forth new experiences, both internal and external.

Time is a contradiction. It seems so long when you're trying to get through each day, but so short when you consider the time you were able to share with your loved one, even if it had been a substantial number of years.

Definitions change.

Alone isn't just a few hours by yourself to read or relax, it is for the rest of your life or an undetermined time.

Silence is not just peace and quiet; it is the deafening sound of your broken heart beating so loudly and yet no one but you can hear it.

One day, things are really good as I fondly remember something silly we used to do, like stopping the car on a desolate dirt road during an evening drive, turning the radio up full blast and dancing in the headlights.

Another day, when things aren't particularly good, I remember that I will sit at the dinner table alone and have no one to share any conversation with.

Expectations are limited to my self-motivation, for no one is "expecting me home at a certain time" to fix a meal; do the laundry; shop' go to bed or even get up at a certain time; and I certainly don't expect anyone to walk through the door after work; take out the garbage; rub my neck or kiss me good-night.

I think the most dramatic realization since my husband died, was that there was no longer anyone in my home and private life to make me feel that I mattered or counted for something.

My personal validation was now gone.

I began to feel that our social life had revolved around my husband because I was no longer invited anywhere with any frequency.

Maybe they invited 'us', because Larry was so vibrant.

Maybe no one really liked me by myself.

It's amazing what thoughts run through your mind when trying to justify a current situation.

It's like the times Larry was late in coming home from work.

"Maybe there was an accident!" "Maybe he doesn't want to come home to me!" "Maybe I haven't kept up my appearance to please him!"

"Maybe I am too fat or nag too much or not enough fun!"

Wow! The power of the mind to make up stories to convince yourself that whatever the reason, it must be your fault.

I remember not too long ago, waking from a dream where I saw Larry and as I drew close, he turned and walked away from me.

I consciously know he wouldn't do that, but my subconscious was having a "field day" with me and for the briefest moment, that vision was an actual consideration in my mind.

Every day, I remind myself of the wonderful times we shared and the happy times when the whole family was together. It would be so very easy to fall into a mental trap where I thought it possible that I was so unlovable, that Larry's dying was the only way he could get away from me, and why was there ever a time I was so prideful and righteous that I thought I had any self-worth?

Depression is such an easy trap to succumb to. Why do I have the right to be happy? I feel so guilty for smiling! Today there was a span of 3 minutes when I didn't think of him. I even had a good nights' sleep and no one pulled on the covers.

There is nothing wrong in seeking counseling during this time. What you're feeling and thinking is normal but sometimes one needs a new perspective and a "sounding board" to vent our emotions and help sort out the new and complex world we now live in.

I find great comfort in prayer. My faith helps keep me grounded, and the knowledge that my God is always with me and I am able to talk to Him, made me feel less alone and abandoned. It was in some of the quietest moments, that I felt the closest to my husband, as if he were residing in my brain and by re-playing a special event, I could almost feel his presence.

I learned a special exercise technique which has been invaluable to me!

I now use this technique over and over again when things get rough and I need to be comforted.

I pick a certain time and place when it was just the two of us.

I find a totally quiet place, close my eyes and literally re-live each moment, in exact detail.

I begin by having a place where Larry would already be present and then envision my entering the room.

I mentally re-create about a 15 minute session and at the end of that time, I must leave the scene, but he must stay.

He cannot come with me and be with me.

Every time I need to feel his presence. I can begin again and return to the place I left him and it begins again.

Choose a special time you remember and do this exercise whenever you feel the need, but relive every minute the way it unfolded, and don't rush. This is your special time to re-connect and although it should be no longer than 15-20 minutes of recalled detail, you must always enter alone and leave alone.

You are alone now in reality; and this must not change, in your exercise of envisionment.

The hardest part of this exercise is finding the quiet time without any possibility of interruptions.
I usually choose the time when I am going to bed. That way I am calm and it is quiet.

Though the first few times you perform this exercise are particularly emotional, it gets more pleasant and easier.

Be careful not to overstay your image time and NEVER forget that you must arrive alone and leave alone.
I haven't done this exercise much in the last 2 years though I always remember every detail of that night and can return whenever I want to.
Sometimes I change the event, though I have a personal favorite and it is filled with the most memorable time just 2 months before Larry's death, when he still had some strength and days of well-being.
I have been able to share this exercise with several people who were going through a particularly difficult time and actually quietly talked them through the event while they had their eyes closed and I was able to watch the healing emotions as they happened.
It was so vivid that I could almost perceive their thoughts during the process.
It is magical what transpires. The human mind is so strong and after completing this exercise, you can see a change has taken place within the individual.
A peace has settled within them and you know that they will carry with them this new knowledge that has the power to help the healing process in the days to come.

For me, it was the first time, in a long time, that I felt I had a purpose all my own and I mattered to someone else.

I've found that the more I am able to help someone else, the more it also helps me.
My life is now different, but here---different is okay.

The reality that I am now a widow and have been left alone is sometimes pretty scary. I was married more than half of my life and I really don't know how to function as a single person anymore.
Everyday is a new experience. Sometimes good and sometimes just awful.
The world has gone through a lot of changes in the last 40 years since I was a single young woman. I was engrossed in a world of being married, raising children and wasn't functioning any longer in a "singles" world.
I lost track of what was involved in being totally independent and making all the decisions without anyone to bounce decisions off of.
Becoming a "single" again is to me, like being thrown ONTO a moving train and not having a map or destination. It is a real culture shock to be sure!!!!
For the longest time I could not go into a restaurant, sit down and order a meal and actually eat it there. I would look around and notice that everyone either was part of a family or had another person with them. I would become so uncomfortable that I would just have my order to go and either eat it in the car or take it home where I was safe from observing eyes.
Now I know that a lot of people eat out by themselves but I haven't arrived at that comfortable place yet and it will be coming upon the ten year anniversary of Larry's death at the end

of May. I don't know where my mindset should be to achieve this and many other things.

I never dwelled upon my own mortality before. There was marriage, raising a family, work and day to day activities.

It wasn't until Larry's death that I began to think about and be concerned as to who would now look after me, should anything happen.

My children were all grown and had their own lives to contend with.

I would not impose on them to appease my concerns.

Then almost six years after Larry passed away, my own health took a startling turn. It was discovered that I was having problems with my blood clotting too much and I developed severe blood clots in both legs from my knees to my liver. In 1986, I experienced two Pulmonary Embolisms within four months.

I had a Stainless Steel implant known as a 'Greenfilter implant' surgically inserted in my Vena Cava. The object was to stop any further blood clots from traveling to my lungs from below the waist. This was very satisfactory and I had no further problems until December of 2005 when I traveled to Germany on a sixteen hour flight for a River Cruise. By the time I arrived in Frankfort, I could not walk any major distance and required a wheelchair. In fact, by the time I reached the ship, after traveling by bus from the airport for another two hours, I was almost unable to walk at all.

I spent almost the entire ten days in my cabin and had to have my meals delivered because walking to the dining room was so much effort and painful.

I did try to go to the city on the first tour, but the guide had to summon a cab to take me to the bus which was literally parked less than one block away. So, I decided to stay on board for the duration.

Sharon J. Hoffman

The friend I was traveling with helped me immensely and without her, I wouldn't have been able to cope by myself.

Makes me appreciate how people with permanent handicaps do the amazing things they do and some do them alone.

Upon returning to my home, I rested and recuperated to return to daily activities----until September of 2006.

I had a scheduled surgical procedure on September 13th and was home recuperating. My daughters had been taking care of me in my home since I was released from the hospital on the 14th.

They would assist me with walking, meals and usual post-operative care.

They returned to their own homes and lives on the 21st of September, leaving me to myself, which was fine.

I was able to do things for myself in slow motion.

I awoke the morning of the 23rd, and was unable to walk. It felt like my legs were actually paralyzed and I couldn't figure out what had happened. I also realized I hadn't gone to the kitchen to get water or food before bedtime the previous evening or gotten up in the night for the bathroom.

I had a certain ritual to perform daily.

Upon rising, I was to walk to the kitchen, get the 'walk about phone' from the charger, get food and water before returning to my bedroom.

Between walks to strengthen and recover my strength, I was to call my friend, here locally; my son in Glendale, Arizona and my daughter in California to report in.

I was barely able to walk to the kitchen to get the phone.

Though only fifty feet down the hall, it took me almost a half hour, with a cane and holding onto the wall while crying out in pain.

I thought I wouldn't make it and yet I knew I had to.

I was terrified of falling and not being able to get up.

With no one but me in the house, I mustered the strength to slowly and deliberately make my way to the phone. Then I realized I had to get back to my chair in the bedroom. I had been sleeping in a lift-chair as I was unable to get in and out of bed by myself.

When I finally made my way to the bedroom, exhausted, I called the doctor. His nurse kept me on the phone, taking my blood pressure and reporting how I was feeling. After about an hour without improvement, she told me to get to urgent care.

How? My thought was that I couldn't do it. I was unable to walk let alone drive and with wrought-iron security gate at my front door, no emergency personnel could get to me without breaking down my door and then having no way to repair it.

I tried to reach my friend who lived locally and to whom I had given a key to my house. I tried several times and even left a message on her answering machine as she wasn't home.

Finally, after a couple of hours she called me back and I told her I needed to get to my Doctor's after hours Urgent Care.

She and her husband arrived and took me to their car in a wheelchair I had. Then they drove me to the Doctor's office.

I signed in and when the nurse saw the pallor of my skin and my current distress, took me into a treatment room quickly.

My doctor came in, took my blood pressure which was now 100/82 and told his nurse to do 'One thing only'! Call 911!

The ambulance arrived and transported me to the hospital where I spent the next two weeks.

Many tests later, it was discovered I had thrown a 3rd Pulmonary Embolism to my lung. I was also anemic and dehydrated.

Doctors were puzzled but immediately thought my recent surgery was the problem, only the severe blood clots in both legs could NOT have manifested so quickly to such a degree.

I remember one of the Doctors saying to me that they had NEVER seen such extensive blood clots before. They said the

Greenfilter implant was full to capacity and no longer able to ward off clots so there would be danger of the clots traveling to my lungs and eventually my heart, which would kill me.

Since the Greenfilter was sewed into my Vena Cava, the only way to replace or insert another was another surgical procedure which would compound my situation with potential life-threatening effects.

I was started on an anticoagulation treatment with injections into my abdomen which soon resulted in hemorrhaging every time I would roll over or attempt to sit up.

I had a lot of time to think about how the blood clots could have manifested so quickly and I finally remembered my trip to Germany and mentioned the incident to the Doctor in charge. It seemed feasible to him but it was never discussed or further mentioned.

(NOTE) Remember this and I will get back to it.

When it was time to be released, there was talk about sending me to a Nursing home as I was not able to care for myself after this incident. The anticoagulation injections had caused a large Seroma (pooling of blood) in my abdomen and the prior healing stitches to open up and these needed packing and bandage dressings every two hours or less for at least the next six weeks.

I didn't know what I was going to do!

I definitely wouldn't consider a Nursing home as with current staffing, it would be impossible for them to attend to my frequent bandaging as it would take a full time nurse for me alone notwithstanding the other patients.

They told me I could not be home alone as; to care for my 5 open wounds required someone to be standing in front of me, able to see from that vantage point, how to clean and bandage my abdomen.

I had wounds that ranged from hip to hip at the lowest bikini line imaginable.

Thank God for my daughter in California! She was able to come for 12 days and care for me in my own home. She had to learn and then improvise methods of care and hygiene from bathing to bandaging.

Then she had to teach me!

After ten days, I learned by being totally reclined in the lift-chair, balancing a mirror between my knees and working backward with packing gauze strips--4x4 gauze pads and tape that wouldn't tear my skin off in removing it, I was able to change my own bandages is just over an hour. That meant I had just about an hour and a half before doing it all over again.

I also had to learn to go to the kitchen and bathroom using the wheelchair.

My daughter put a cooler by my chair filled with water bottles.

Food tasted terrible to me and I was unable to cook so I was reduced to eating jars of baby food and granola bars.

Large boxes of medical supplies were placed on the floor close to my chair.

Recuperating has been a long long process and it is now almost eight months since I was released from the hospital and although my wounds are outwardly healed, there is still internal healing which is taking longer. I have no idea how long it will continue.

Upon my release, I continued to question as to an answer as to why I tend to produce so many more clots than anyone else.

Could there be a blood test to determine the origin?

(Remember the NOTE at the top of the page? Here is the rest of that story!)

A blood test was finally performed at my insistence.

What you don't know is: I was adopted at 3 weeks old.

Sharon J. Hoffman

No medical records or un-identifying information had ever been made available. So, everything was an unknown.

The blood test came back indicating I have a Protein 'C' deficiency.

I also have a Protein 'S' deficiency. I also have too much Fibrin in my body. All this encourages a hyper-clotting disorder.

I will be on an anticoagulant for the rest of my life and there is no real prognosis for me.

The Doctors in the hospital when asked about my prognosis, told me that they couldn''t tell me when or even "IF" I would survive this event, as so few people have both deficiencies and no real studies have been recorded due to the intense degree of clotting that I have.

Well, isn't that a great kettle of fish????

Maybe now you see why I have reason to question my mortality to the degree that I do.